Table of Contents

"Tips and Tricks to Boost a Woman's Sex Drive"

Introduction

Discuss the importance of a healthy sex drive for overall well-being.

Overview of the factors affecting a woman's libido (physical, emotional, psychological).

Introduce the book's purpose: providing actionable tips and tricks to boost a woman's sex drive.

Setting the tone: empowering, respectful, and supportive.

Chapter 1: Understanding Female Sexual Desire

Anatomy and physiology of female sexual response. Common

myths and misconceptions about women's libido.

How age, hormones, and life stages (e.g., pregnancy, menopause) affect sex drive. Importance

of self-awareness and communication in addressing sexual needs.

Chapter 2: Physical Health and Its Impact on Libido

* Nutrition: Foods that support a healthy sex drive (e.g., aphrodisiacs, vitamins).
* Exercise: How physical activity can enhance sexual desire.
* Sleep: The role of rest in maintaining energy levels and libido.
* Hormonal balance: The impact of thyroid, oestrogen, and testosterone on sex drive.

Chapter 3: Mental and Emotional Health

* Stress and its effects on libido: How to manage stress for a better sex life.
* The impact of anxiety and depression on sexual desire.
* Building self-esteem and body confidence.
* The role of mental health therapy in improving sex drive.

Chapter 4: Relationship Dyna

Communication: How talking openly with your partner can enhance intimacy.
* Addressing common relationship issues that affect sexual desire (e.g., conflict, resentment).
* Building emotional intimacy to boost physical desire.
* Role of foreplay and affection in increasing libido.

Chapter 5: Lifestyle Changes for Boosting Libido

* Being available for intimacy in busy schedules.
* The impact of alcohol, smoking, and substance use on sexual health.
* Mindfulness and relaxation techniques for enhancing sexual desire.
* How setting the mood (lighting, music, ambiance) can affect libido.

Chapter 6: Exploring New Experiences

* The importance of variety in sexual relationships: keeping things fresh and exciting.
* Exploring fantasies and desires safely with your partner.
* Using sex toys and other aids to enhance sexual experiences.
* Communication around trying new things: ensuring both partners are comfortable.

Chapter 7: Natural Supplements and Remedies

- Overview of natural herbs and supplements that can support libido (e.g., maca root, ginseng).
- Risks and benefits: what to consider before trying natural remedies.
- How to incorporate supplements into your lifestyle for maximum effect.
- Consultations with health professionals: when to seek advice before using natural remedies.

Chapter 8: Medical Solutions for Low Libido

- When to seek medical advice: recognizing symptoms of underlying health issues.
- Prescription medications that can help with libido (e.g., hormone replacement therapy).
- Counseling and therapy: working with professionals to address deeper issues.
- Navigating side effects: how to balance medical treatments with natural approaches.

Chapter 9: Myths, Misconceptions, and Social Influences

- Debunking common myths about female sexual desire.
- The impact of societal expectations on women's sex drive.
- How media portrayal of sex can distort expectations.Encouraging a healthy, positive view of sexuality.

Chapter 10: Long-Term Strategies for Maintaining a Healthy Sex Drive

- Building habits that support sustained sexual health and desire.
- Nurturing your relationship to keep the sexual connection strong over time.
- Planning for different life stages: how to adapt your strategies as you age.
- Celebrating sexuality as part of overall health and well-being.

Conclusion

- Recap of key takeaways.
- Encouragement to embrace a healthy, satisfying sexual life.
- Final words of support and empowerment.

Introduction

Sexual health is an integral part of overall well-being. For many women, maintaining a healthy sex drive is about more than just physical pleasure; it is deeply connected to emotional and mental health, intimacy in relationships, and even self-confidence. However, it is not uncommon for a woman's libido to fluctuate due to several factors such as stress, hormonal changes, or relationship dynamics.

A decline in sexual desire can feel confusing and frustrating, especially when there is a lack of information and support on how to address it. This book is here to change that by providing practical tips and tricks that any woman can implement to reignite her passion and boost her libido.

The Importance of a Healthy Sex Drive

A healthy sex drive is often a reflection of balance in a woman's life. It can indicate that her body is functioning well, that she feels emotionally connected in her relationships, and that she is confident in her own skin. When libido declines, it is often a signal that something is off, whether it is a health issue, stress, or an emotional challenge.

Sexual satisfaction has a ripple effect on other areas of life. When a woman feels connected and fulfilled in her intimate relationships, it can enhance her self-esteem, improve her mood, and even positively impact her physical health. Conversely, a diminished sex drive can lead to feelings of frustration, distance in relationships, and even a decline in general well-being.

Factors Affecting a Woman's Libido

Women's sexual desire is complex, influenced by a mix of physical, emotional, psychological, and even social factors. Hormonal fluctuations during menstruation, pregnancy, and menopause play a significant role, as do health conditions such as thyroid imbalances or chronic illnesses. Emotional factors like stress, anxiety, and depression can also dampen a woman's libido.

Relationship dynamics are another key factor. Feeling emotionally disconnected from a partner, unresolved conflicts, or even boredom in a long-term relationship can reduce sexual desire. Similarly, lifestyle factors such as sleep deprivation, poor nutrition, and lack of exercise can contribute to a low libido.

Understanding these factors is the first step in addressing low libido. By identifying what might be contributing to a decline in sexual desire, women can take targeted steps to address those issues, whether through lifestyle changes, relationship adjustments, or seeking medical advice.

The Purpose of This Book

This book is designed to empower women with knowledge and practical strategies to boost their sex drive. Each chapter covers a different aspect of sexual health, from physical wellness to emotional well-being, relationship dynamics, and lifestyle changes. The goal is to provide a comprehensive approach that addresses the numerous factors affecting libido and offers actionable tips to make positive changes.

Whether you are looking to reignite your passion, improve your relationship, or simply feel more connected to your body, this book is for you. Sexual desire is not something that should be ignored or dismissed—it is a vital part of who you are. By taking steps to enhance your libido, you are not only improving your sex life but also nurturing your overall well-being.

So, let us begin this journey together. Through self-awareness, understanding, and the application of practical tips, you can reclaim your sexual desire and enjoy a fulfilling, vibrant sex life.

This introduction provides a comprehensive overview of the book's purpose and the importance of addressing sexual health. I will move on to Chapter 1: Understanding Female Sexual Desire next.

Chapter 1: Understanding Female Sexual Desire

Sexual desire is a complex, multifaceted aspect of human experience, and for women, it involves a delicate interplay of biological, psychological, and emotional factors. Understanding the basics of female sexual response and the influences that can enhance or dampen libido is essential to addressing any challenges in this area. In this chapter, we will explore the anatomy and physiology of female sexual desire, debunk common myths, and discuss how age, hormones, and life stages can impact a woman's libido.

Anatomy and Physiology of Female Sexual Response

At the heart of female sexual desire is the body's intricate sexual response system. The female body is designed for sexual pleasure, with various parts working together to create arousal, excitement, and satisfaction. Understanding this anatomy can help women become more in tune with their bodies and better communicate their needs.

1. **The Brain: The Control Center of Desire**
   - Sexual desire often begins in the brain. Thoughts, memories, fantasies, and emotional connections play a significant role in triggering arousal. The brain releases chemicals like dopamine, which enhance pleasure and desire, and oxytocin, which fosters emotional bonding. When a woman is emotionally connected with her partner or feels relaxed and confident, her brain is more likely to initiate the desire for sexual intimacy.
2. **The Clitoris: A Key Player in Sexual Pleasure**
   - The clitoris is the most sensitive part of a woman's sexual anatomy, containing thousands of nerve endings. Unlike male genitalia, the clitoris exists solely for pleasure, making it a crucial element in female arousal. Understanding and embracing the importance of clitoral stimulation can enhance sexual experiences for many women.
3. **The Vagina and Vulva: Physical Responses to Arousal**
   - During arousal, the vagina and vulva undergo changes, including increased blood flow, lubrication, and expansion. These physiological responses help prepare the body for sexual activity and increase sensitivity to touch, making sexual experiences more pleasurable.
4. **Hormones: The Unsung Heroes**
   - Hormones like estrogen, testosterone, and progesterone play critical roles in regulating sexual desire. These hormones fluctuate throughout a woman's life, particularly during menstruation, pregnancy, and menopause, affecting libido at various stages. For instance, testosterone, although often associated with men, is vital for women's sexual desire, while estrogen helps maintain vaginal lubrication and elasticity.

Debunking Myths and Misconceptions

Despite advancements in sexual education, many myths about female sexuality still persist. These misconceptions can lead to unrealistic expectations, feelings of inadequacy, or confusion about what's "normal." Let's address some of the most common myths:

5. **Myth: Women Should Always Be Ready for Sex**
   - Reality: Sexual desire is not constant, and it's perfectly normal for libido to fluctuate. Stress, fatigue, emotional well-being, and physical health all impact

sexual desire. It's important to listen to your body and not feel pressured to be "in the mood" all the time.

6. **Myth: Men Have Higher Sex Drives Than Women**
   - o Reality: Libido is highly individual, and many women have robust sex drives. However, societal expectations and stereotypes often lead women to downplay their desire. It's essential to recognize that sexual desire varies from person to person and is not strictly determined by gender.

7. **Myth: A Woman's Libido Naturally Declines with Age**
   - o Reality: While hormonal changes during menopause can affect libido, many women continue to experience strong sexual desire well into their later years. With the right approach to health and well-being, age doesn't have to diminish sexual satisfaction.

The Impact of Age, Hormones, and Life Stages on Libido

A woman's sexual desire is not static; it changes over time due to hormonal fluctuations, life events, and even personal growth. Understanding these changes can help women navigate periods of low libido with greater self-compassion and knowledge.

8. **Menstruation and Libido**
   - o Hormonal changes throughout the menstrual cycle can influence sexual desire. Many women report increased libido during ovulation when oestrogen and testosterone levels peak. On the other hand, premenstrual syndrome (PMS) or menstrual discomfort can dampen desire.

9. **Pregnancy and Postpartum Changes**
   - o During pregnancy, increased blood flow to the pelvic area and heightened hormone levels can boost libido for some women. However, fatigue, nausea, and body changes may have the opposite effect for others. Postpartum, fluctuating hormones, sleep deprivation, and the demands of caring for a newborn can all impact a woman's desire for intimacy.

10. **Menopause and Beyond**
    - o Menopause brings about significant hormonal changes, particularly a decline in oestrogen and testosterone. These changes can lead to vaginal dryness, reduced sensitivity, and a drop in libido. However, many women find that with proper management of symptoms, they can continue to enjoy a healthy sex life. Hormone replacement therapy (HRT), vaginal moisturizers, and lifestyle adjustments can all help maintain sexual desire during and after menopause.

11. **Life Events and Stressors**
    - o Major life events, such as starting a new job, moving, or experiencing loss, can have a profound impact on sexual desire. Stress, in particular, is a major libido killer. When the body is in a state of high stress, it prioritizes survival over reproduction, often leading to a significant drop in sexual desire. Learning to manage stress through relaxation techniques, therapy, or lifestyle changes can help restore balance.

The Importance of Self-Awareness and Communication

Self-awareness is a powerful tool in enhancing sexual desire. Understanding your own body needs, and preferences can help you take control of your sexual health. Regularly checking in with yourself—both physically and emotionally—can reveal patterns in your libido and help identify what might be influencing it.

Communication is equally important. Open, honest discussions with your partner about your needs, desires, and any challenges you're facing can strengthen your connection and improve your sexual relationship. By being proactive in addressing issues, you can foster a healthier, more satisfying sex life.

This chapter outlines the foundational knowledge necessary for understanding female sexual desire.

Chapter 2: Physical Health and Its Impact on Libido

Physical health is a key factor in maintaining a strong sex drive. When the body is healthy and balanced, it's easier to feel energized and in the mood for intimacy. On the other hand, when physical well-being is compromised, sexual desire can take a hit. In this chapter, we will explore how nutrition, exercise, sleep, and hormonal balance contribute to a healthy libido, and offer practical tips for optimizing these areas of your life.

Nutrition: Foods That Support a Healthy Sex Drive

The saying "you are what you eat" holds true when it comes to sexual health. Certain foods can boost energy levels, balance hormones, and even enhance sexual desire. On the flip side, poor nutrition can lead to fatigue, low energy, and hormonal imbalances that diminish libido. Here are some foods that can support a healthy sex drive:

12. Aphrodisiacs: Foods That Stimulate Desire
- Aphrodisiacs are foods believed to increase sexual desire and performance. While their effects may vary from person to person, some popular aphrodisiac foods include:
  - **Dark Chocolate:** Rich in phenylethylamine, a compound that stimulates the release of feel-good hormones, dark chocolate can enhance mood and increase sexual desire.
  - **Oysters:** High in zinc, which is crucial for the production of testosterone, oysters have long been considered a potent aphrodisiac.
  - **Avocados:** Loaded with healthy fats and vitamin E, avocados support hormone production and promote blood flow, which can enhance arousal.

- **Chili Peppers:** Capsaicin, the compound that gives chili peppers their heat, can increase heart rate and trigger the release of endorphins, both of which can boost libido.

13. Nutrient-Rich Foods for Hormonal Balance

- Hormones play a central role in regulating sexual desire, and the right nutrients can help keep them balanced. Foods that support hormone health include:
  - **Leafy Greens (e.g., spinach, kale):** High in magnesium, which helps regulate cortisol (the stress hormone) and promotes healthy blood flow.
  - **Fatty Fish (e.g., salmon, mackerel):** Packed with omega-3 fatty acids, which support heart health and reduce inflammation, leading to improved circulation and sexual health.
  - **Nuts and Seeds (e.g., almonds, flaxseeds):** Rich in essential fatty acids and zinc, which help balance hormone levels and boost libido.

14. The Impact of Processed Foods and Sugar

- While whole, nutrient-dense foods support a healthy sex drive, processed foods and excessive sugar can have the opposite effect. High-sugar diets can lead to insulin resistance, which affects hormone levels and energy. Additionally, processed foods often lack the nutrients needed for hormonal balance, leading to fatigue and a reduced libido.

Exercise: How Physical Activity Can Enhance Sexual Desire

Regular exercise is one of the most effective ways to boost libido. Physical activity improves circulation, enhances mood, reduces stress, and increases energy levels—all of which contribute to a healthy sex drive. Here's how exercise can benefit your sexual health:

15. Improved Blood Flow

- Exercise helps improve cardiovascular health, which in turn enhances blood flow throughout the body, including to the genital area. This increased circulation can lead to better arousal and heightened sensitivity during sexual activity.

16. Stress Reduction and Mood Enhancement

- Exercise triggers the release of endorphins, the body's natural "feel-good" chemicals. Regular physical activity can help reduce stress, anxiety, and depression, all of which are common contributors to low libido. When stress levels are managed, it's easier to feel relaxed and in the mood for intimacy.

17. Increased Energy and Stamina

- Regular exercise boosts energy levels and improves overall fitness, which can lead to more satisfying sexual experiences. When you feel strong and energized, you're more likely to engage in and enjoy physical intimacy.

18. Body Confidence

- Exercise can improve body image and self-esteem, which are important factors in sexual desire. When you feel good about your body, you're more likely to feel confident and comfortable in intimate situations.

19. Best Types of Exercise for Sexual Health

- While all forms of exercise are beneficial, certain types can be particularly helpful for boosting libido:

- **Cardiovascular Exercise (e.g., running, cycling):** Supports heart health and improves circulation.
- **Strength Training (e.g., weight lifting):** Builds muscle, increases endurance, and enhances body confidence.
- **Yoga and Pilates:** Improve flexibility, reduce stress, and help connect the mind and body, which can enhance sexual awareness.

Sleep: The Role of Rest in Maintaining Energy Levels and Libido

Sleep is a critical component of physical health, and it plays a major role in sexual desire. When the body is well-rested, it's more likely to have the energy and hormonal balance needed to maintain a healthy libido. However, chronic sleep deprivation can lead to fatigue, irritability, and decreased sexual desire.

20. How Sleep Affects Hormones
- Sleep is essential for regulating hormones that influence libido, including testosterone, oestrogen, and cortisol. Poor sleep can disrupt these hormones, leading to reduced sexual desire. For example, inadequate sleep can cause a drop in testosterone levels, which are important for maintaining sexual desire in both men and women.

21. The Link Between Sleep Quality and Sexual Satisfaction
- Research has shown that people who get sufficient, high-quality sleep report higher levels of sexual satisfaction. A good night's rest can improve mood, increase energy levels, and enhance overall well-being, all of which contribute to a healthier sex drive.

22. Tips for Improving Sleep
- Prioritize a regular sleep schedule by going to bed and waking up at the same time each day.
- Create a relaxing bedtime routine that helps signal to your body that it's time to wind down (e.g., reading, taking a warm bath, or practicing mindfulness).
- Avoid heavy meals, caffeine, and electronic devices before bed, as these can interfere with sleep quality.

Hormonal Balance: The Impact of Thyroid, Oestrogen, and Testosterone on Sex Drive

Hormonal imbalances are one of the most common culprits behind a decline in libido. The body's hormonal system is complex, and even small changes in hormone levels can have a big impact on sexual desire. Here's a closer look at how key hormones affect libido:

23. Thyroid Hormones
- The thyroid gland produces hormones that regulate metabolism and energy levels. An underactive thyroid (hypothyroidism) can lead to fatigue, weight gain, and a decrease in libido. If you suspect a thyroid issue may be affecting your sex drive, it's important to consult with a healthcare provider for testing and treatment.

24. Oestrogen
- Oestrogen is a primary female sex hormone that plays a significant role in sexual health. It helps maintain vaginal lubrication, elasticity, and blood flow, all of which are important for sexual arousal and comfort. Oestrogen levels

fluctuate throughout a woman's life, particularly during menstruation, pregnancy, and menopause, and these fluctuations can affect libido.

25. Testosterone
- o Often associated with male sexual health, testosterone is also crucial for women's libido. Low testosterone levels can lead to a decrease in sexual desire and energy. Certain conditions, such as polycystic ovary syndrome (PCOS) or menopause, can impact testosterone levels, so it's important to monitor hormonal health and seek treatment if necessary.

26. Balancing Hormones Naturally
- o While medical treatment may be necessary for some hormonal imbalances, there are natural ways to support hormonal health:
    - **Manage Stress:** Chronic stress can disrupt hormone levels, so stress management techniques like meditation, yoga, and deep breathing can help.
    - **Eat a Balanced Diet:** A nutrient-rich diet supports hormone production and balance. Focus on whole foods, healthy fats, and adequate protein.
    - **Exercise Regularly:** Physical activity helps regulate hormones and promotes overall well-being.
    - **Get Enough Sleep:** As mentioned earlier, sleep is crucial for hormonal regulation.

This chapter highlights the importance of physical health in maintaining a healthy libido, offering practical advice on nutrition, exercise, sleep, and hormonal balance.

Chapter 3: Mental and Emotional Health

Mental and emotional well-being are deeply intertwined with sexual desire. Stress, anxiety, depression, and self-esteem issues can all have a significant impact on libido. Understanding how these factors affect sexual desire is essential for making positive changes that can help restore a healthy sex drive. In this chapter, we will explore how mental and emotional health influence libido and offer strategies for managing stress, building confidence, and seeking support when needed.

Stress and Its Effects on Libido

Stress is one of the most common culprits behind a diminished sex drive. When life becomes overwhelming, the body shifts into survival mode, prioritizing essential functions over reproduction and pleasure. High levels of stress can lead to a cascade of effects that ultimately reduce libido.

27. The Physiological Impact of Stress

- o When the body is under stress, it releases cortisol, the stress hormone, which can interfere with the production of sex hormones like oestrogen and testosterone. Chronic stress can disrupt the delicate hormonal balance necessary for maintaining sexual desire. Additionally, stress can lead to physical symptoms such as tension, headaches, and fatigue, all of which can diminish interest in sex.

28. Mental and Emotional Exhaustion

- o Stress can take a toll on mental and emotional health, leading to feelings of exhaustion, irritability, and detachment. When the mind is preoccupied with worries or overwhelmed by daily responsibilities, it can be difficult to feel relaxed or in the mood for intimacy. Emotional stressors, such as relationship conflicts or financial concerns, can also contribute to a decline in libido.

29. Managing Stress for a Better Sex Life

- o Learning to manage stress is essential for maintaining a healthy sex drive. Here are some strategies that can help:
  - **Mindfulness and Meditation:** Practicing mindfulness and meditation can help reduce stress by promoting relaxation and present-moment awareness. These techniques can also improve emotional connection with a partner, enhancing intimacy.
  - **Exercise:** Physical activity is a powerful stress-reliever. Regular exercise helps release endorphins, improve mood, and reduce tension, all of which can positively impact libido.
  - **Prioritize Self-Care:** Taking time for self-care activities, such as reading, taking a bath, or spending time in nature, can help reduce stress and improve overall well-being.
  - **Set Boundaries:** Learning to say no and setting boundaries with work, family, and social obligations can reduce feelings of overwhelm and create more space for relaxation and intimacy.

The Impact of Anxiety and Depression on Sexual Desire

Anxiety and depression are two of the most common mental health conditions, and both can have a profound impact on sexual desire. The symptoms of these conditions can interfere with sexual interest, arousal, and satisfaction, making it difficult to enjoy intimacy.

30. Anxiety and Its Effects on Libido

- o Anxiety can manifest in many forms, from general worry and nervousness to panic attacks and obsessive thoughts. For those who struggle with anxiety, sexual activity can feel overwhelming or even frightening. Anxiety can lead to physical symptoms such as rapid heartbeat, muscle tension, and shortness of breath, which can make it difficult to relax and enjoy intimacy.
- o Additionally, anxiety can create a cycle of negative thinking. Worries about sexual performance, body image, or relationship dynamics can fuel further anxiety, making it challenging to engage in sexual activity.

31. Depression and Its Effects on Libido

- o Depression often leads to a loss of interest in activities that once brought pleasure, including sex. Feelings of sadness, hopelessness, and low energy can make it difficult to muster the motivation for intimacy. Depression can also affect self-esteem and body image, further reducing sexual desire.

- Physical symptoms of depression, such as fatigue and changes in appetite or sleep patterns, can also contribute to a decline in libido. Additionally, some medications used to treat depression, such as selective serotonin reuptake inhibitors (SSRIs), can have side effects that affect sexual desire and function.

32. Seeking Support for Mental Health Challenges

- If anxiety or depression is affecting your libido, it's important to seek support from a mental health professional. Therapy, counselling, and medication can all be effective in managing these conditions and improving overall well-being. Cognitive-behavioural therapy (CBT), in particular, is a popular approach for addressing anxiety and depression, as it helps individuals challenge negative thought patterns and develop healthier coping strategies.
- Support groups and peer networks can also provide valuable emotional support. Talking with others who understand what you're going through can help reduce feelings of isolation and provide new perspectives on managing mental health and sexual desire.

Building Self-Esteem and Body Confidence

A healthy sense of self-esteem and body confidence is essential for a satisfying sex life. When a woman feels good about herself, she is more likely to feel comfortable and confident in intimate situations. Conversely, low self-esteem and negative body image can lead to anxiety, self-consciousness, and a reduced desire for sexual activity.

33. The Link Between Body Image and Sexual Desire

- Body image plays a significant role in sexual confidence. Women who struggle with body dissatisfaction may avoid sexual activity due to feelings of embarrassment or shame. These negative feelings can create a barrier to intimacy, making it difficult to enjoy sexual experiences.
- On the other hand, women who feel confident in their bodies are more likely to engage in and enjoy sexual activity. Positive body image is associated with greater sexual satisfaction, increased desire, and improved overall well-being.

34. Strategies for Building Self-Esteem and Body Confidence

- **Practice Self-Compassion:** Treat yourself with kindness and compassion, especially when it comes to your body. Instead of focusing on perceived flaws, try to appreciate your body for all that it does for you.
- **Challenge Negative Thoughts:** Pay attention to negative self-talk and challenge those thoughts. Ask yourself if they are realistic or if they are based on societal pressures or unrealistic expectations.
- **Surround Yourself with Positivity:** Surround yourself with people, media, and environments that promote body positivity and self-acceptance. Avoid sources of negativity or comparison that may contribute to low self-esteem.
- **Take Care of Your Body:** Engaging in activities that make you feel good, such as exercise, healthy eating, and grooming, can improve body confidence and self-esteem.

The Role of Mental Health Therapy in Improving Sex Drive

Therapy can be a powerful tool for addressing the mental and emotional factors that affect libido. Whether you're dealing with stress, anxiety, depression, or self-esteem issues, working with a therapist can help you gain insight into your feelings and develop strategies for improving your sexual desire.

35. **Types of Therapy for Sexual Health**
    - **Cognitive-Behavioural Therapy (CBT):** CBT focuses on identifying and changing negative thought patterns that can contribute to anxiety, depression, and low self-esteem. By addressing these underlying issues, CBT can help improve sexual desire and satisfaction.
    - **Sex Therapy:** Sex therapy is a specialized form of therapy that focuses on sexual concerns and challenges. A sex therapist can help you explore issues related to libido, sexual function, and relationship dynamics, offering guidance and support for improving your sex life.
    - **Couples Therapy:** If relationship issues are contributing to a decline in libido, couples therapy can help improve communication, resolve conflicts, and rebuild emotional intimacy.
36. **When to Seek Professional Help**
    - If you've noticed a significant decline in your libido and it's affecting your quality of life or relationships, it may be time to seek professional help. A mental health professional can help you explore the underlying causes of low libido and develop a personalized plan for improving your sexual health.

This chapter emphasizes the importance of mental and emotional well-being in maintaining a healthy libido.

Chapter 4: Relationship Dynamics

The dynamics of a relationship play a crucial role in shaping sexual desire. When a relationship is strong, characterized by open communication, mutual respect, and emotional intimacy, sexual desire tends to flourish. However, when there are unresolved conflicts, poor communication, or emotional distance, libido can wane. This chapter explores how various aspects of relationship dynamics affect sexual desire and offers practical strategies for improving intimacy and connection with your partner.

Communication: The Foundation of Intimacy

Communication is the cornerstone of a healthy sexual relationship. Open, honest discussions about needs, desires, and boundaries can enhance intimacy and ensure that both partners feel understood and valued. Unfortunately, many couples struggle to talk about sex, often due to embarrassment, fear of rejection, or simply not knowing how to start the conversation.

37. **Why Communication Matters**
    - Effective communication fosters trust and emotional closeness, which are essential for a healthy sex life. When partners feel safe and connected, they are more likely to express their desires and engage in fulfilling sexual experiences. Conversely, when communication breaks down, misunderstandings and resentment can build, leading to a decline in sexual desire.
38. **How to Improve Communication About Sex**
    - **Start the Conversation:** Choose a relaxed, private setting to talk about your sexual relationship. Begin by expressing your feelings and asking open-ended questions to encourage dialogue. For example, you might say, "I've been thinking about our sex life and wanted to talk about how we can make it even better."
    - **Listen Actively:** Give your partner your full attention when they speak, and avoid interrupting. Reflect on what they're saying and ask clarifying questions if needed. Active listening helps both partners feel heard and understood.
    - **Be Honest and Compassionate:** Share your thoughts and feelings openly, but do so with kindness and sensitivity. Avoid blaming or criticizing your partner, and instead focus on expressing your own experiences and needs.
    - **Practice Patience:** Talking about sex can be challenging, especially if it's a new topic for your relationship. Be patient with each other, and recognize that it may take time to build comfort and openness in these conversations.

Addressing Common Relationship Issues That Affect Libido

All relationships face challenges from time to time, and these challenges can have a direct impact on sexual desire. Whether it's stress from daily life, unresolved conflicts, or a loss of emotional connection, these issues can create barriers to intimacy. Addressing these problems head-on is essential for maintaining a healthy sex drive.

39. **Stress and Its Impact on the Relationship**
    - External stressors, such as work pressures, financial worries, or family responsibilities, can spill over into a relationship and affect sexual desire. When both partners are stressed, they may feel too exhausted or preoccupied to engage in intimacy. Additionally, stress can lead to irritability and tension, making it harder to connect emotionally and physically.
    - **Solution:** Identify the sources of stress and work together to manage them. This might involve delegating responsibilities, setting boundaries, or finding ways to relax and recharge as a couple. Prioritizing time for each other, even during stressful periods, can help maintain the emotional connection that supports a healthy sex life.
40. **Unresolved Conflicts and Resentment**
    - Unresolved conflicts can create emotional distance and resentment, both of which can dampen sexual desire. When conflicts go unaddressed, they can fester and lead to a breakdown in communication and intimacy. Resentment, in particular, can create a barrier to physical closeness, as it often stems from feelings of hurt or betrayal.
    - **Solution:** Address conflicts as they arise, rather than letting them build up. Practice conflict resolution skills, such as active listening, compromise, and

finding common ground. Couples therapy can also be beneficial in helping partners navigate difficult issues and rebuild trust and connection.

41. Loss of Emotional Connection

- o Emotional intimacy is the bedrock of a healthy sexual relationship. When partners feel emotionally connected, they are more likely to desire physical closeness. However, if that connection weakens over time, sexual desire can diminish as well. This loss of connection can occur for various reasons, such as growing apart, lack of quality time together, or becoming too focused on individual pursuits.
- o **Solution:** Make a conscious effort to reconnect emotionally. This might involve spending more quality time together, engaging in shared activities, or simply talking more openly about your feelings and experiences. Rebuilding emotional intimacy can reignite sexual desire and strengthen your relationship.

Building Emotional Intimacy to Boost Physical Desire

Emotional intimacy and physical desire are closely linked. When partners feel emotionally close, they are more likely to experience sexual desire. Building and maintaining emotional intimacy requires ongoing effort, but the rewards in terms of relationship satisfaction and sexual fulfilment are well worth it.

42. Cultivating Emotional Closeness

- o Emotional closeness is about feeling deeply connected to your partner on a personal level. It involves understanding each other's needs, values, and experiences, and being there to support each other through life's ups and downs. To cultivate this closeness:
    - **Share Vulnerabilities:** Open up about your fears, hopes, and insecurities. Sharing these deeper aspects of yourself can strengthen your bond and make you feel more connected.
    - **Show Appreciation:** Regularly express gratitude and appreciation for your partner. Acknowledging the positive aspects of your relationship reinforces emotional connection.
    - **Be Present:** Focus on your partner when you're together. Put away distractions, such as phones or laptops, and engage fully in your time together.

43. The Role of Affection in Enhancing Libido

- o Physical affection, such as hugging, kissing, and cuddling, plays a significant role in maintaining emotional and sexual intimacy. These small acts of affection can increase feelings of love and connection, making it easier to transition into sexual activity.
    - **Increase Non-Sexual Touch:** Incorporate more non-sexual touch into your daily routine. This might include holding hands, giving massages, or simply sitting close to each other. These gestures can enhance feelings of closeness and support a healthy libido.
    - **Make Time for Intimacy:** Set aside dedicated time for intimacy, even if it's just a few minutes each day. This could involve sharing a kiss before leaving for work, having a date night, or spending time in bed together before sleep.

The Role of Foreplay and Affection in Increasing Libido

Foreplay is not just a prelude to sex; it's an essential part of building sexual desire and enhancing intimacy. Engaging in extended foreplay allows both partners to relax, connect, and become fully aroused, leading to more satisfying sexual experiences.

44. **Why Foreplay Matters**
    - Foreplay helps set the stage for sexual activity by increasing physical and emotional arousal. It allows time for both partners to become fully engaged in the experience, which can lead to stronger desire and more pleasurable sex. Additionally, foreplay can enhance communication, as it often involves verbal and non-verbal cues about what feels good and what each partner enjoys.
45. **Incorporating More Foreplay Into Your Relationship**
    - **Slow Down:** Take your time during foreplay. Rather than rushing to intercourse, focus on exploring each other's bodies, kissing, touching, and enjoying the build-up of desire.
    - **Experiment:** Try new techniques or activities during foreplay to keep things exciting. This could involve using massage oils, experimenting with different types of touch, or incorporating verbal expressions of desire.
    - **Prioritize Mutual Pleasure:** Make foreplay a mutually enjoyable experience. Pay attention to your partner's reactions and communicate openly about what feels good. This mutual focus on pleasure can enhance the connection and make the experience more satisfying for both partners.

This chapter emphasizes the importance of mental and emotional well-being in maintaining a healthy libido.

Chapter 5: Lifestyle Changes for Boosting Libido

Lifestyle choices have a profound impact on sexual desire. The way you manage your time, your habits, and even your environment can either enhance or diminish libido. In this chapter, we'll explore how lifestyle changes such as prioritizing intimacy, addressing substance use, practicing mindfulness, and setting the right mood can boost your sex drive and improve your overall sexual health.

Making Time for Intimacy in Busy Schedules

In today's fast-paced world, it's easy to become overwhelmed by responsibilities and obligations, leaving little time or energy for intimacy. However, prioritizing your relationship and making time for sexual activity is essential for maintaining a healthy libido. When intimacy becomes a regular part of your routine, it's more likely to flourish.

46. **The Importance of Scheduling Intimacy**

- While spontaneity is often idealized, scheduling intimacy can be just as important, especially in long-term relationships. By setting aside dedicated time for sexual activity, you ensure that it remains a priority in your busy life. This practice can help prevent the gradual decline of sexual desire that often accompanies busy schedules.

47. Tips for Making Time for Intimacy

- **Plan Date Nights:** Regular date nights are a great way to maintain emotional and physical connection. Plan activities that you both enjoy and that foster closeness, whether it's going out for dinner, taking a walk, or watching a movie together.
- **Set Boundaries:** Establish clear boundaries between work, personal life, and relationship time. Avoid letting work or other responsibilities encroach on the time you've set aside for your partner.
- **Create Rituals:** Develop small daily or weekly rituals that promote intimacy. This could be something as simple as sharing a morning coffee, spending a few minutes cuddling before bed, or giving each other a massage.

48. Overcoming Obstacles to Scheduled Intimacy

- Scheduling intimacy doesn't mean it has to feel forced or routine. Keep the excitement alive by varying the activities and environments, and by being open to spontaneous moments of connection when they arise. Remember, the goal is to create opportunities for intimacy, not to turn it into a chore.

The Impact of Alcohol, Smoking, and Substance Use on Sexual Health

Substance use, including alcohol, smoking, and recreational drugs, can have a significant impact on sexual desire and performance. While some substances may temporarily lower inhibitions or increase arousal, their long-term effects can be detrimental to sexual health.

49. Alcohol and Libido

- Alcohol is often associated with social and sexual behavior, as it can reduce inhibitions and increase confidence. However, excessive alcohol consumption can have the opposite effect, leading to decreased libido and sexual performance issues. Chronic alcohol use can also lead to hormonal imbalances and impair the body's ability to respond to sexual stimuli.

50. Smoking and Its Effects on Sexual Desire

- Smoking has a negative impact on overall health, and sexual health is no exception. Nicotine and other chemicals in cigarettes can reduce blood flow to the genitals, leading to difficulties with arousal and orgasm. Smoking is also associated with decreased libido and can contribute to a decline in sexual satisfaction over time.

51. The Role of Recreational Drugs

- Recreational drugs, such as marijuana, cocaine, and ecstasy, can alter perception and increase arousal temporarily. However, these substances can also disrupt normal brain function, lead to dependence, and have negative effects on sexual desire and performance. Long-term use of recreational drugs can result in decreased libido, sexual dysfunction, and relationship issues.

52. Strategies for Reducing or Eliminating Substance Use

- o **Seek Support:** If you're struggling with substance use, seek support from a healthcare provider, therapist, or support group. Addressing substance use issues can lead to significant improvements in sexual health and overall well-being.
- o **Practice Moderation:** If you choose to consume alcohol, do so in moderation. Avoid using substances as a way to cope with stress or enhance sexual experiences, as this can lead to dependence and long-term sexual health issues.
- o **Focus on Healthy Habits:** Replace substance use with healthier habits that support sexual health, such as regular exercise, a balanced diet, and stress management techniques.

Mindfulness and Relaxation Techniques for Enhancing Sexual Desire

Mindfulness and relaxation techniques can have a powerful impact on sexual desire by helping to reduce stress, increase self-awareness, and enhance emotional and physical connection with your partner. These practices encourage you to be fully present in the moment, which can lead to more fulfilling sexual experiences.

53. The Benefits of Mindfulness for Sexual Health
- o Mindfulness involves paying attention to the present moment without judgment. In the context of sexual health, mindfulness can help you become more attuned to your body's sensations and your partner's cues, leading to a deeper connection and greater sexual satisfaction. Mindfulness can also reduce anxiety and negative self-talk, which are common barriers to a healthy libido.

54. Relaxation Techniques for Reducing Stress
- o Stress is one of the biggest inhibitors of sexual desire. Incorporating relaxation techniques into your daily routine can help lower stress levels and create a more conducive environment for intimacy. Techniques such as deep breathing, progressive muscle relaxation, and meditation can calm the mind and body, making it easier to focus on pleasure.

55. Practicing Mindfulness During Intimacy
- o **Focus on Sensations:** During sexual activity, pay close attention to the physical sensations in your body. Notice the texture of your partner's skin, the rhythm of your breathing, and the warmth of touch. By staying present, you can enhance the pleasure and connection you feel.
- o **Let Go of Expectations:** Release any expectations or goals for the sexual experience, such as reaching orgasm or performing in a certain way. Instead, focus on enjoying the experience and connecting with your partner.
- o **Communicate Openly:** Mindful communication involves expressing your desires and needs clearly and listening to your partner without judgment. This openness fosters trust and intimacy, which can enhance sexual desire.

How Setting the Mood Can Affect Libido

The environment in which sexual activity takes place can have a significant impact on desire. Creating a space that feels comfortable, relaxing, and conducive to intimacy can enhance arousal and make sexual experiences more enjoyable.

56. The Role of Ambiance in Sexual Desire
  - o   The ambiance of a room, including lighting, music, and scents, can influence your mood and sexual desire. A cluttered, noisy, or uncomfortable environment can be distracting and reduce libido, while a well-curated space can help you feel more relaxed and in the mood for intimacy.

57. Tips for Setting the Mood
  - o   **Lighting:** Soft, warm lighting can create a more intimate and relaxing atmosphere. Consider using candles, dimmable lights, or soft lamps to set the right mood.
  - o   **Music:** Music can enhance the emotional and sensory experience of intimacy. Choose music that you both enjoy and that helps you feel connected and aroused.
  - o   **Scents:** Aromatherapy can be a powerful tool for enhancing libido. Scents like lavender, jasmine, and ylang-ylang are known for their relaxing and aphrodisiac properties. Use scented candles, essential oils, or incense to create a soothing and sensual environment.
  - o   **Comfort:** Ensure that your space is physically comfortable, with soft bedding, pillows, and a pleasant temperature. The more comfortable you feel, the easier it is to relax and focus on the experience.

This chapter has provided practical insights into how lifestyle changes can positively impact sexual desire.

Chapter 6: Exploring New Experiences

Variety is often described as the spice of life, and this is especially true in sexual relationships. Introducing new experiences, whether through exploring fantasies, trying new activities, or incorporating toys and aids, can help keep sexual desire alive and vibrant. In this chapter, we'll explore the importance of variety, how to safely explore fantasies and desires, and tips for introducing new elements into your sexual relationship to enhance pleasure and intimacy.

The Importance of Variety in Sexual Relationships

Over time, even the most passionate relationships can experience a decline in sexual excitement. This is a natural part of being in a long-term relationship, but it doesn't have to mean the end of a fulfilling sex life. By introducing variety and novelty into your sexual experiences, you can reignite the spark and maintain a strong sexual connection with your partner.

58. Why Variety Matters

- o Routine and predictability can lead to boredom in any aspect of life, including sex. When sexual activity becomes too routine, it can start to feel like a chore rather than an exciting and pleasurable experience. Introducing variety helps break the monotony and keeps things fresh and exciting, which can enhance desire and satisfaction.

59. Ways to Introduce Variety

- o **Try New Positions:** Experimenting with different sexual positions can bring a new dimension to your physical connection. Each position offers a unique experience in terms of sensation, intimacy, and pleasure.
- o **Explore Different Settings:** Changing the location of your sexual encounters can add excitement. Whether it's a different room in your home, a romantic getaway, or an outdoor setting, new environments can stimulate desire.
- o **Incorporate Role-Playing:** Role-playing allows you to step out of your usual roles and explore different personas. This can be a fun and creative way to add variety and excitement to your sex life.

60. Maintaining Variety Over Time

- o Variety doesn't have to mean constantly seeking out new experiences; it can also involve revisiting and alternating between activities that you and your partner enjoy. The key is to stay open to trying new things and to communicate openly about what works for both of you.

Exploring Fantasies and Desires Safely With Your Partner

Fantasies and desires are a natural part of human sexuality, and exploring them with a partner can lead to deeper intimacy and enhanced pleasure. However, it's important to approach this exploration with care and communication to ensure that both partners feel comfortable and respected.

61. The Role of Fantasies in Sexual Desire

- o Fantasies can be a powerful tool for enhancing sexual desire. They allow individuals to explore their deepest desires and curiosities in a safe and imaginative way. Sharing fantasies with a partner can strengthen your connection and lead to new, exciting experiences.

62. How to Safely Explore Fantasies

- o **Communicate Openly:** Before exploring any fantasies, have an open and honest conversation with your partner. Discuss your desires, boundaries, and any concerns you might have. It's important that both partners feel heard and respected.
- o **Establish Boundaries:** Set clear boundaries for what is and isn't comfortable for each of you. This ensures that the experience remains positive and enjoyable for both partners.
- o **Start Slowly:** If you're new to exploring fantasies together, start with something simple and gradually build up to more complex scenarios. This allows you to gauge each other's comfort levels and adjust as needed.
- o **Use Safe Words:** If you're engaging in role-play or any activity that involves power dynamics or intense emotions, establish a safe word that either partner can use to pause or stop the activity if they feel uncomfortable.

63. When Not to Act on Fantasies

- o It's important to recognize that not all fantasies need to be acted upon. Some fantasies may be better left in the realm of imagination, especially if they could harm your relationship or involve risks that you're not willing to take. Always prioritize mutual respect and consent.

Using Sex Toys and Other Aids to Enhance Sexual Experiences

Sex toys and aids can add a new dimension to sexual experiences, offering opportunities for enhanced pleasure and exploration. Whether you're introducing toys for the first time or looking to expand your collection, there are plenty of options to suit different preferences and comfort levels.

64. Benefits of Incorporating Sex Toys
- o **Increased Pleasure:** Sex toys can stimulate areas of the body in ways that may not be possible through manual or oral stimulation alone. They can also help intensify orgasms and provide new sensations.
- o **Enhancing Intimacy:** Using toys together can be a bonding experience, as it involves trust, communication, and mutual exploration. It can also be a way to introduce variety into your sex life.
- o **Solo and Partner Use:** Toys can be used both during solo play and with a partner, offering flexibility in how you incorporate them into your sexual routine.

65. Choosing the Right Toys
- o **Consider Your Preferences:** Think about what types of stimulation you and your partner enjoy, whether it's clitoral, vaginal, anal, or a combination. Choose toys that align with those preferences.
- o **Start Simple:** If you're new to using sex toys, start with something simple, such as a small vibrator or a set of handcuffs. As you become more comfortable, you can explore more advanced toys.
- o **Focus on Quality:** Invest in high-quality toys made from body-safe materials. Look for products that are easy to clean and maintain, and that have positive reviews from other users.

66. Introducing Toys to Your Relationship
- o **Communicate First:** Talk to your partner about your interest in using toys and discuss any concerns or preferences they might have. This conversation can help ensure that both partners are on the same page.
- o **Use Toys as a Complement:** Rather than replacing traditional sexual activity, use toys as a complement to enhance your experiences. This approach can help ease any concerns about toys diminishing the role of your partner in your sexual relationship.
- o **Experiment Together:** Spend time exploring the toy together, discovering what feels good and how it can enhance your sexual connection. This mutual exploration can be a fun and intimate experience.

Communication Around Trying New Things: Ensuring Comfort and Consent

Introducing new experiences into your sex life can be exciting, but it's essential to prioritize communication, comfort, and consent. Both partners should feel safe and respected when trying something new, and open dialogue is key to achieving this.

67. **The Importance of Mutual Consent**
    o   Consent is the foundation of any healthy sexual relationship. Before trying anything new, ensure that both you and your partner are fully on board. Consent should be enthusiastic, informed, and ongoing, meaning that either partner can withdraw consent at any time if they feel uncomfortable.
68. **Tips for Discussing New Experiences**
    o   **Choose the Right Time:** Have conversations about new experiences in a relaxed, non-sexual setting where both partners feel comfortable. This allows for an open discussion without the pressure of the moment.
    o   **Be Open and Honest:** Share your desires and interests with your partner, but also be open to hearing theirs. Approach the conversation with curiosity rather than judgment.
    o   **Respect Boundaries:** If your partner is not comfortable with a particular idea, respect their boundaries without pressure or coercion. Focus on finding mutually enjoyable activities that you both feel excited about.
69. **Navigating Disagreements**
    o   It's natural for partners to have different comfort levels when it comes to trying new things. If you disagree on an idea, use it as an opportunity to learn more about each other's preferences and find a compromise that works for both of you. Remember, the goal is to enhance your sexual connection, not create tension or discomfort.

This chapter has explored how introducing variety, exploring fantasies, and using toys can enhance sexual desire and intimacy.

Chapter 7: Natural Supplements and Remedies

For centuries, people have turned to natural remedies and supplements to enhance sexual desire and overall sexual health. While modern medicine offers various treatments for low libido, many women prefer to explore natural options first. In this chapter, we will explore some of the most popular natural supplements and remedies that are believed to support libido, discuss their potential benefits and risks, and provide guidance on how to incorporate them safely into your lifestyle.

Overview of Natural Herbs and Supplements for Libido

Natural herbs and supplements have been used for generations to boost libido, balance hormones, and improve sexual health. These remedies are often derived from plants and minerals and are believed to work by enhancing blood flow, balancing hormones, and reducing stress.

70. Maca Root

- **What It Is:** Maca is a root vegetable native to the Andes Mountains of Peru. It has been used traditionally for its energy-boosting and aphrodisiac properties.
- **How It Works:** Maca is believed to help balance hormones, increase energy levels, and improve sexual function. It's often used by women experiencing low libido due to hormonal imbalances, such as those related to menopause or stress.
- **How to Use It:** Maca is available in powder form, capsules, or extracts. It can be added to smoothies, baked goods, or taken as a supplement. The typical dosage ranges from 1,500 to 3,000 mg per day.
- **Potential Side Effects:** Maca is generally considered safe, but some people may experience digestive issues, such as bloating or stomach discomfort, especially when taking high doses.

71. Ginseng

- **What It Is:** Ginseng is a root that has been used in traditional Chinese medicine for centuries to enhance energy, reduce stress, and improve sexual function.
- **How It Works:** Ginseng is believed to increase nitric oxide production, which improves blood flow and can enhance arousal and sexual pleasure. It also has adaptogenic properties, meaning it helps the body adapt to stress, which can indirectly support libido.
- **How to Use It:** Ginseng is available in capsules, teas, and extracts. The typical dosage ranges from 200 to 400 mg per day. It's important to use ginseng in moderation, as excessive consumption can lead to side effects.
- **Potential Side Effects:** Some people may experience insomnia, headaches, or gastrointestinal issues when taking ginseng. It may also interact with certain medications, so it's important to consult with a healthcare provider before use.

72. Tribulus Terrestris

- **What It Is:** Tribulus Terrestris is a plant commonly used in traditional medicine to boost libido and support reproductive health.
- **How It Works:** Tribulus is believed to increase levels of certain hormones, including oestrogen, which can help improve libido in women. It's often used to address sexual dysfunction and enhance sexual satisfaction.
- **How to Use It:** Tribulus is available in capsule or powder form. The typical dosage ranges from 250 to 1,500 mg per day. It's important to start with a lower dose and gradually increase to assess tolerance.
- **Potential Side Effects:** Tribulus is generally well-tolerated, but some people may experience stomach upset, restlessness, or changes in mood.

73. Ashwagandha

- **What It Is:** Ashwagandha is an adaptogenic herb commonly used in Ayurvedic medicine to reduce stress, boost energy, and improve sexual health.
- **How It Works:** Ashwagandha is believed to reduce cortisol levels (the stress hormone) and enhance overall well-being. By reducing stress and anxiety, it can help improve libido and sexual function.

- o **How to Use It:** Ashwagandha is available in capsules, powders, and extracts. The typical dosage ranges from 300 to 600 mg per day. It's often taken with food to reduce the risk of digestive discomfort.
  - o **Potential Side Effects:** Ashwagandha is generally safe, but some people may experience drowsiness, digestive upset, or changes in mood. It's important to use it under the guidance of a healthcare provider, especially if you're taking other medications.

74. L-Arginine

- o **What It Is:** L-Arginine is an amino acid that plays a key role in the production of nitric oxide, a compound that helps relax blood vessels and improve blood flow.
  - o **How It Works:** By increasing nitric oxide levels, L-Arginine can enhance blood flow to the genital area, improving arousal and sexual function. It's often used by individuals experiencing sexual dysfunction related to poor circulation.
  - o **How to Use It:** L-Arginine is available in capsules, powders, and tablets. The typical dosage ranges from 2,000 to 6,000 mg per day, taken in divided doses. It's important to start with a lower dose to assess tolerance.
  - o **Potential Side Effects:** Some people may experience gastrointestinal issues, such as diarrhoea or nausea, when taking L-Arginine. It may also interact with certain medications, such as blood pressure medications, so it's important to consult with a healthcare provider before use.

Risks and Benefits: What to Consider Before Trying Natural Remedies

While natural supplements and remedies can offer potential benefits for libido, it's important to consider the risks and consult with a healthcare provider before starting any new supplement. Here are some factors to keep in mind:

75. Quality and Purity

- o Not all supplements are created equal. The quality and purity of natural supplements can vary widely between brands. Look for products that are third-party tested for quality and safety and choose reputable brands that have positive reviews and transparent sourcing practices.

76. Potential Interactions with Medications

- o Natural supplements can interact with prescription and over-the-counter medications, potentially leading to adverse effects. For example, ginseng may interact with blood thinners, and L-Arginine may affect blood pressure medications. Always consult with a healthcare provider before adding any new supplement to your routine, especially if you're taking other medications or have underlying health conditions.

77. Individual Responses

- o The effectiveness of natural remedies can vary from person to person. While some individuals may experience significant improvements in libido, others may not notice much of a difference. It's important to manage your expectations and be open to trying different approaches if needed.

78. Long-Term Use

- o While many natural supplements are considered safe for short-term use, the long-term effects are less well-studied. It's important to take breaks from supplements and avoid using them in excessively high doses. Regular check-ins with your healthcare provider can help ensure that your supplement regimen remains safe and effective.

How to Incorporate Supplements Into Your Lifestyle for Maximum Effect

Incorporating natural supplements into your lifestyle can be an effective way to support libido, but it's important to do so in a thoughtful and informed manner. Here are some tips for getting the most out of natural remedies:

79. Start Slowly
   - Begin with a lower dose of any new supplement to assess how your body responds. Gradually increase the dosage as needed, but avoid exceeding the recommended amount. This approach helps minimize the risk of side effects and allows you to gauge the supplement's effectiveness.

80. Maintain a Balanced Diet
   - Supplements should complement, not replace, a healthy diet. Focus on eating a balanced diet rich in whole foods, including fruits, vegetables, lean proteins, and healthy fats. A nutrient-rich diet provides the foundation for overall health and can enhance the effects of natural supplements.

81. Combine with Other Healthy Habits
   - Supplements work best when combined with other healthy lifestyle habits. Regular exercise, stress management techniques, adequate sleep, and open communication with your partner can all contribute to improved sexual health and desire.

82. Track Your Progress
   - Keep a journal or notes on how you feel after taking supplements. Note any changes in your libido, mood, energy levels, and overall well-being. Tracking your progress can help you determine which supplements are most effective for you and whether any adjustments are needed.

83. Consult a Healthcare Provider
   - Regular consultations with a healthcare provider can help ensure that your supplement regimen is safe and effective. Your provider can offer personalized advice, monitor your progress, and help you navigate any potential interactions or side effects.

This chapter has provided an overview of natural supplements and remedies that can support libido, along with tips for safely incorporating them into your lifestyle.

Chapter 8: Medical Solutions for Low Libido

While lifestyle changes and natural remedies can be effective in boosting libido for many women, there are times when medical intervention may be necessary. Low libido can sometimes be a symptom of underlying health issues that require professional evaluation and treatment. In this chapter, we will explore when to seek medical advice, the role of prescription medications, and other medical treatments available for addressing low libido.

When to Seek Medical Advice: Recognizing Symptoms of Underlying Health Issues

Low libido can be caused by a wide range of factors, including hormonal imbalances, chronic health conditions, and certain medications. If you've tried lifestyle changes and natural remedies without significant improvement, or if your low libido is accompanied by other concerning symptoms, it may be time to seek medical advice.

84. **Persistent or Severe Low Libido**
    o   If your low libido is persistent, severe, or affecting your quality of life or relationships, it's important to consult with a healthcare provider. A thorough evaluation can help identify any underlying medical conditions that may be contributing to the problem.

85. **Hormonal Imbalances**
    o   Hormonal imbalances, such as those related to thyroid function, oestrogen, or testosterone levels, can have a significant impact on libido. Symptoms of hormonal imbalances may include irregular menstrual cycles, weight changes, fatigue, and mood swings. If you suspect a hormonal issue, your healthcare provider can perform blood tests to assess hormone levels and recommend appropriate treatments.

86. **Chronic Health Conditions**
    o   Conditions such as diabetes, cardiovascular disease, and chronic pain can affect sexual desire and function. Additionally, mental health conditions like depression and anxiety can lead to a decline in libido. If you have a chronic health condition that you suspect is affecting your sex drive, it's important to discuss this with your healthcare provider.

87. **Side Effects of Medications**
    o   Certain medications, including antidepressants, antihypertensives, and hormonal contraceptives, can have side effects that reduce libido. If you've noticed a decline in sexual desire after starting a new medication, talk to your healthcare provider about alternative treatments or adjustments to your current regimen.

Prescription Medications That Can Help With Libido

When lifestyle changes and natural remedies aren't enough, prescription medications may be an option for addressing low libido. Several medications are available that can help boost sexual desire, particularly in cases where hormonal imbalances or other medical issues are contributing to the problem.

88. **Hormone Replacement Therapy (HRT)**
    o   **What It Is:** Hormone Replacement Therapy involves supplementing the body with hormones, such as oestrogen, progesterone, or testosterone, to balance hormonal levels.

- How It Works: HRT is often used to address symptoms of menopause, such as hot flashes, vaginal dryness, and low libido, by restoring hormonal balance. For women experiencing low libido due to menopause or other hormonal imbalances, HRT can be an effective treatment.
  - Considerations: HRT is not suitable for everyone, and it's important to discuss the risks and benefits with your healthcare provider. Potential side effects include an increased risk of blood clots, stroke, and certain types of cancer.

89. Flibanserin (Addyi)

  - What It Is: Flibanserin, sold under the brand name Addyi, is a prescription medication specifically approved for the treatment of hypoactive sexual desire disorder (HSDD) in premenopausal women.
  - How It Works: Flibanserin works by affecting neurotransmitters in the brain, such as serotonin, dopamine, and norepinephrine, to increase sexual desire. It's typically taken daily, and results may take several weeks to become noticeable.
  - Considerations: Flibanserin can cause side effects such as dizziness, fatigue, and nausea. It also has restrictions on alcohol consumption due to the risk of severe low blood pressure and fainting. It's important to discuss potential risks and benefits with your healthcare provider before starting this medication.

90. Bremelanotide (Vyleesi)

  - What It Is: Bremelanotide, sold under the brand name Vyleesi, is an injectable medication used to treat HSDD in premenopausal women.
  - How It Works: Bremelanotide is a melanocortin receptor agonist that is thought to work by activating pathways in the brain that are involved in sexual desire. It is typically administered as a self-injection about 45 minutes before anticipated sexual activity.
  - Considerations: Common side effects of Bremelanotide include nausea, headache, and flushing. As with any medication, it is important to discuss potential risks and benefits with your healthcare provider.

91. Testosterone Therapy

  - What It Is: Testosterone therapy involves supplementing the body with testosterone, a hormone that plays a key role in sexual desire for both men and women.
  - How It Works: Low testosterone levels can contribute to low libido in women, particularly those who have undergone menopause. Testosterone therapy can help restore libido by balancing hormone levels.
  - Considerations: Testosterone therapy is typically prescribed off-label for women, and it's important to work closely with a healthcare provider to monitor hormone levels and minimize the risk of side effects, such as acne, hair growth, or voice changes.

Counselling and Therapy: Working with Professionals to Address Deeper Issues

In addition to medications, counselling and therapy can be effective in addressing the psychological and emotional factors that contribute to low libido. Whether you're dealing with relationship issues, mental health concerns, or stress, working with a trained professional can provide valuable support and guidance.

92. Sex Therapy

- o **What It Is:** Sex therapy is a specialized form of therapy that focuses on addressing sexual concerns and improving sexual health. It can help individuals and couples explore the emotional, psychological, and relational aspects of low libido.
- o **How It Works:** A sex therapist works with you to identify the underlying causes of low libido, such as stress, trauma, or relationship issues, and develop strategies for improving sexual desire and satisfaction. This may involve techniques such as cognitive-behavioural therapy (CBT), mindfulness practices, and communication exercises.
- o **Considerations:** Sex therapy can be beneficial for both individuals and couples. It is important to find a qualified and experienced therapist who specializes in sexual health.

93. Cognitive-Behavioural Therapy (CBT)

- o **What It Is:** Cognitive-behavioural therapy is a type of talk therapy that focuses on identifying and changing negative thought patterns and behaviours that contribute to low libido.
- o **How It Works:** CBT can help individuals challenge and reframe negative beliefs about sex, improve self-esteem, and develop healthier coping mechanisms for dealing with stress and anxiety. This can lead to an increase in sexual desire and overall well-being.
- o **Considerations:** CBT is a structured, goal-oriented therapy that typically involves regular sessions with a trained therapist. It can be an effective treatment for those dealing with mental health issues, such as anxiety or depression, that are affecting libido.

94. Couples Therapy

- o **What It Is:** Couples therapy is a form of therapy that focuses on improving communication and resolving conflicts within a relationship. It can be particularly helpful for couples experiencing sexual difficulties, including low libido.
- o **How It Works:** A couples therapist works with both partners to identify the underlying issues that may be contributing to sexual dissatisfaction, such as unresolved conflicts, poor communication, or emotional distance. Therapy sessions may involve exercises and techniques to improve intimacy, rebuild trust, and enhance sexual connection.
- o **Considerations:** Couples therapy can be an effective way to address relationship dynamics that are affecting libido. It's important to choose a therapist who is experienced in working with sexual health issues.

Navigating Side Effects: How to Balance Medical Treatments With Natural Approaches

When using medical treatments for low libido, it's important to be aware of potential side effects and how to manage them. Balancing medical treatments with natural approaches can help you achieve the best possible outcome while minimizing risks.

95. Monitoring and Managing Side Effects

- o If you experience side effects from prescription medications or therapies, it's important to communicate with your healthcare provider. They may be able to adjust your dosage, switch medications, or recommend additional treatments to alleviate side effects.

96. Incorporating Natural Remedies

o   Natural remedies, such as herbs, supplements, and lifestyle changes, can complement medical treatments and help reduce the risk of side effects. For example, mindfulness practices can reduce stress and anxiety, which may help mitigate some of the side effects of medication.

97. Regular Check-Ins with Your Healthcare Provider

o   Regular follow-up appointments with your healthcare provider are essential for monitoring your progress and making any necessary adjustments to your treatment plan. This ensures that your approach to managing low libido remains safe, effective, and aligned with your overall health goals.

This chapter has provided an overview of medical solutions for low libido, including when to seek medical advice, the role of prescription medications, and the benefits of therapy.

Chapter 9: Myths, Misconceptions, and Social Influences

Sexual desire, especially in women, has long been a topic shrouded in myths and misconceptions. These false beliefs are often perpetuated by societal expectations, cultural norms, and media portrayals, leading to confusion and unrealistic expectations about what is "normal" when it comes to libido. In this chapter, we will debunk common myths about female sexual desire, examine the impact of societal influences, and explore how to foster a healthy, positive view of sexuality.

Debunking Common Myths About Female Sexual Desire

Myths about female libido have been around for centuries, often rooted in outdated or incorrect understandings of women's bodies and sexuality. These myths can contribute to feelings of shame, inadequacy, or confusion. Let us address some of the most pervasive myths and set the record straight.

98. Myth: Women Should Always Be in the Mood for Sex

o   **Reality:** Sexual desire naturally fluctuates due to a variety of factors, including stress, hormones, relationship dynamics, and overall health. It's completely normal for women (and men) to experience periods of higher or lower libido. The idea that women should always be in the mood is unrealistic and can lead to unnecessary pressure and stress.

99. Myth: Low Libido Means You Do not Love Your Partner

- o **Reality:** Sexual desire is not always linked to love or affection for a partner. Many factors, including physical health, mental well-being, and external stressors, can affect libido independently of one's feelings for their partner. It is important to communicate openly about these issues without assuming that low libido reflects a lack of love.

100. **Myth: Men Have Higher Sex Drives Than Women**
   - o **Reality:** While societal stereotypes often portray men as having higher sex drives, libido is highly individual and not strictly determined by gender. Many women have strong, consistent sex drives, and many men experience fluctuations in libido. The key is recognizing and honouring everyone's unique sexual needs and desires.
101. **Myth: A Decline in Libido Is Inevitable with Age**
   - o **Reality:** While hormonal changes during menopause can affect libido, many women continue to enjoy a healthy and satisfying sex life well into their later years. With the right approach to health, including hormone management, communication, and lifestyle adjustments, age does not have to be a barrier to sexual satisfaction.
102. **Myth: Sexual Desire Peaks in Youth**
   - o **Reality:** The belief that sexual desire peaks in youth and declines afterward is another misconception. Many women find that their sexual confidence and enjoyment increase with age, as they become more comfortable with their bodies and their desires. Sexual satisfaction is not limited to any specific age group.

The Impact of Societal Expectations on Women's Sex Drive

Society often places unrealistic expectations on women when it comes to sexual desire, contributing to feelings of inadequacy or pressure. These expectations are shaped by cultural norms, gender roles, and the media, all of which can influence how women perceive their own libido.

103. **Cultural Norms and Gender Roles**
   - o Cultural norms and traditional gender roles often dictate how women "should" behave sexually. For example, women may be expected to be modest and restrained, while men are encouraged to be sexually assertive. These stereotypes can lead women to suppress their desires or feel guilty about expressing them, which can negatively impact libido.
104. **The Pressure to Perform**
   - o Women are often subjected to societal pressure to meet certain sexual standards, whether it is maintaining a high libido, being a "perfect" partner, or adhering to specific beauty standards. This pressure can create anxiety and stress, which are known inhibitors of sexual desire. It is important to recognize that sexual experiences should be about mutual pleasure and connection, not meeting external expectations.
105. **The Double Standard**
   - o The double standard around sexuality often celebrates male sexual conquests while shaming women for expressing their desires. This double standard can lead to internalized shame and confusion about what is

"acceptable" behaviour for women, further complicating their relationship with their own sexuality.

106. **Challenging Societal Expectations**
   - o Challenging societal expectations requires a conscious effort to embrace your own desires and reject the stereotypes that limit sexual expression. It is important to surround yourself with supportive voices and to engage in open conversations about sexuality that promote a healthy, balanced view of sexual desire.

How Media Portrayal of Sex Can Distort Expectations

The media plays a significant role in shaping societal views on sex and sexual desire. However, the portrayal of sex in movies, television, and advertising is often unrealistic and can lead to distorted expectations about what a healthy sex life should look like.

107. **The Idealized Image of Sex**
   - o Media often presents an idealized version of sex, where encounters are always passionate, spontaneous, and flawless. These portrayals can create unrealistic expectations about sexual performance and satisfaction, leading to disappointment when real-life experiences do not match up.
108. **The Overemphasis on Youth and Appearance**
   - o Media often emphasizes youth and physical appearance as central to sexual desirability, overlooking the diverse experiences and preferences that exist across different ages, body types, and life stages. This narrow portrayal can contribute to body image issues and the belief that only certain people are "worthy" of sexual satisfaction.
109. **The Lack of Realistic Representation**
   - o Many media portrayals of sex fail to represent the diversity of sexual experiences, including different sexual orientations, preferences, and life circumstances. This lack of representation can make some individuals feel alienated or abnormal when their desires or experiences differ from what is commonly depicted.
110. **Fostering a Healthy Media Literacy**
   - o Developing media literacy involves critically analysing the messages presented in media and recognizing their influence on your perceptions of sex and desire. By becoming aware of these influences, you can set more realistic expectations for your own sexual experiences and embrace a more authentic and personal view of sexuality.

Encouraging a Healthy, Positive View of Sexuality

Fostering a healthy and positive view of sexuality is essential for maintaining a satisfying and fulfilling sex life. This involves rejecting harmful myths and stereotypes, embracing your unique desires, and creating an environment that supports sexual well-being.

111. **Embrace Your Individuality**
   - o Sexuality is deeply personal, and what works for one person may not work for another. Embrace your own desires, preferences, and experiences without comparing yourself to others or adhering to societal standards. Recognizing

and accepting your individuality can lead to greater sexual satisfaction and self-confidence.

112. **Open Communication**
   - Open and honest communication with your partner is key to maintaining a healthy sexual relationship. Discuss your desires, boundaries, and any concerns you may have. This openness fosters trust and intimacy, which can enhance your overall sexual experience.
113. **Seek Out Positive Influences**
   - Surround yourself with positive influences that support a healthy view of sexuality. This might include reading books or articles that celebrate diverse sexual experiences, engaging with supportive communities, or seeking guidance from a therapist or counsellor who specializes in sexual health.
114. **Prioritize Self-Care**
   - Taking care of your mental, emotional, and physical health is essential for maintaining a positive view of sexuality. Prioritize self-care practices that reduce stress, boost confidence, and enhance your overall well-being.

Chapter 10: Long-Term Strategies for Maintaining a Healthy Sex Drive

Maintaining a healthy sex drive over the long term requires a holistic approach that encompasses physical health, emotional well-being, and relationship dynamics. As life circumstances change, so too can libido, and it's important to adopt sustainable practices that support sexual health through all stages of life. In this chapter, we'll explore strategies for building habits that support sustained sexual desire, nurturing your relationship, and adapting to different life stages with confidence and grace.

Building Habits That Support Sustained Sexual Health and Desire

Developing and maintaining healthy habits is key to supporting long-term sexual desire. These habits can help ensure that your body and mind remain in optimal condition for enjoying a fulfilling sex life.

115. **Prioritize Physical Health**
   - **Nutrition:** A balanced diet rich in whole foods, healthy fats, lean proteins, and plenty of fruits and vegetables supports overall health, including sexual function. Nutrient-rich foods help maintain hormonal balance, boost energy levels, and support a healthy libido.
   - **Exercise:** Regular physical activity improves circulation, increases energy levels, and reduces stress, all of which are important for maintaining sexual desire. Incorporate a mix of cardiovascular exercises, strength training, and flexibility exercises like yoga to support overall well-being.

- o **Sleep:** Quality sleep is essential for hormonal balance and energy. Aim for 7-9 hours of restful sleep each night to support both your physical and emotional health.

116. **Manage Stress Effectively**
   - o Stress is one of the most significant inhibitors of sexual desire. Develop stress management techniques that work for you, whether it's mindfulness meditation, deep breathing exercises, or engaging in hobbies that help you relax. Reducing stress can help maintain a healthy libido over the long term.

117. **Stay Connected to Your Body**
   - o Regularly check in with your body to understand how you're feeling both physically and emotionally. Pay attention to signs of stress, fatigue, or hormonal changes, and address them proactively. Practices like mindfulness, yoga, and regular physical check-ups can help you stay connected to your body's needs.

118. **Foster Emotional Well-Being**
   - o Emotional health is closely linked to sexual desire. Engage in activities that boost your mood and self-esteem, such as spending time with loved ones, pursuing creative outlets, or practicing gratitude. Taking care of your mental health can help sustain a healthy libido.

Nurturing Your Relationship to Keep the Sexual Connection Strong

A strong, healthy relationship is foundational to maintaining sexual desire over time. Nurturing emotional intimacy, practicing good communication, and keeping the sexual spark alive are all essential components of a satisfying sexual relationship.

119. **Cultivate Emotional Intimacy**
   - o Emotional intimacy involves sharing your thoughts, feelings, and experiences with your partner in a way that deepens your connection. Regularly spend quality time together, engage in meaningful conversations, and support each other through life's challenges. Emotional closeness often translates into physical desire, so investing in your relationship is key to maintaining a strong sexual connection.

120. **Practice Open Communication**
   - o Communication is crucial for a healthy sex life. Regularly check in with your partner about your sexual relationship—discuss what's working, what you'd like to try, and any concerns you may have. Open communication helps ensure that both partners feel understood, valued, and satisfied.

121. **Keep the Spark Alive**
   - o As relationships progress, it's natural for sexual desire to fluctuate. To keep the spark alive, make an effort to introduce variety and excitement into your sexual experiences. This might involve trying new activities, exploring fantasies, or simply making more time for intimacy. Keep the focus on mutual pleasure and connection.

122. **Resolve Conflicts Proactively**
   - o Unresolved conflicts can create emotional distance and reduce sexual desire. Address any issues that arise in your relationship with honesty and compassion. Seeking couples therapy or counselling can also be beneficial if conflicts are affecting your sexual connection.

Planning for Different Life Stages: How to Adapt Your Strategies Over Time

Sexual desire can change throughout life due to factors such as aging, hormonal changes, and life transitions. Adapting your approach to sexual health as you move through different stages of life can help you maintain a satisfying sex drive.

123. **Understanding the Impact of Aging**
     - As women age, hormonal changes, particularly during menopause, can affect libido. These changes might include vaginal dryness, reduced sensitivity, or fluctuations in sexual desire. However, many women continue to enjoy a fulfilling sex life well into their later years. Hormone replacement therapy (HRT), vaginal moisturizers, and regular sexual activity can help mitigate some of the effects of aging.

124. **Adapting to Life Transitions**
     - Major life transitions, such as pregnancy, childbirth, and menopause, can all impact sexual desire. During these times, it's important to be patient with yourself and your partner, and to communicate openly about any changes in your sexual needs or preferences. Adjusting your sexual routine to accommodate these changes can help maintain intimacy and satisfaction.

125. **Embracing Sexuality at Every Age**
     - Sexuality is a lifelong aspect of well-being, and it's important to embrace your sexual desires and needs at every stage of life. Whether you're in your 20s, 40s, or 60s, your sexual health is an important part of your overall health. Continue to explore, communicate, and prioritize your sexual well-being as you age.

126. **Seeking Professional Support When Needed**
     - If you experience significant changes in libido that are affecting your quality of life, it may be helpful to seek professional support. A healthcare provider, sex therapist, or counsellor can offer guidance and treatment options to help you navigate the challenges of different life stages.

Celebrating Sexuality as Part of Overall Health and Well-Being

Sexuality is an integral part of who you are, and maintaining a healthy libido is about more than just physical pleasure—it's about embracing your desires, nurturing your relationships, and supporting your overall well-being. By prioritizing your sexual health and adopting sustainable strategies, you can enjoy a vibrant and satisfying sex life throughout your life.

127. **Embrace Your Sexuality**
     - Celebrate your sexuality as a natural and important part of your identity. Embrace your desires, explore your preferences, and engage in sexual activities that bring you joy and satisfaction.

128. **Integrate Sexual Health into Your Self-Care Routine**
     - Include sexual health as part of your overall self-care routine. Just as you care for your physical, mental, and emotional health, make time to nurture your sexual well-being. This holistic approach ensures that all aspects of your health are aligned and balanced.

129. **Stay Open to Growth and Change**

- o Sexuality is dynamic, and it's natural for desires and preferences to evolve over time. Stay open to growth and change and continue to explore new ways to enhance your sexual health and satisfaction.

This final chapter has provided long-term strategies for maintaining a healthy sex drive, including building sustainable habits, nurturing relationships, and adapting to life changes.